Y0-BVG-102

AN
AURAL
ATLAS

Published Exclusively for the Medical Profession by
AURALGAN RESEARCH DIVISION
NEW YORK, N. Y., U. S. A.

Copyrighted in United States, Canada, and under International and Pan American Copyright Conventions.

ALL RIGHTS RESERVED

This book is protected by copyright. No part of it may be duplicated or reproduced in any manner without written permission from the publisher.

Copyright 1946 By

AURALGAN RESEARCH DIVISION

NEW YORK, N. Y., U. S. A.

Printed in U.S.A.

Edited By

SAMUEL J. KOPETZKY, M.D., F.A.C.S.

Directing Otolaryngologist, New York Polyclinic Medical School & Hospital

RALPH ALMOUR, M.D., F.A.C.S.

Professor of Otolaryngology, New York Polyclinic Medical School & Hospital

JULIUS BELL, M.D., F.A.C.S.

Instructor in Otolaryngology, New York Polyclinic Medical School & Hospital

MURRAY B. GORDON, M.D., F.A.C.P.

Professor of Clinical Pediatrics, Long Island College of Medicine

ILLUSTRATORS

PLATES I, II, III, IV   ALFRED FEINBERG

ALL OTHER ILLUSTRATIONS   MISS EVE MADSEN

INDEX

INDEX

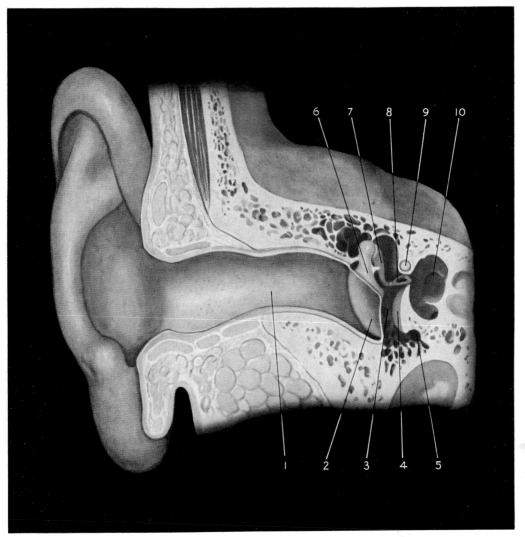

PLATE I

©1946 - AURALGAN - OTOSMOSAN

Frontal Section Through Tympanic Cavity

(1) External Auditory Canal – (2) Tympanic Membrane
(3) Middle Ear – (4) Promontory – (5) Niche of
Round Window – (6) Malleus – (7) Incus – (8) Stapes
(9) Facial Nerve – (10) Vestibule

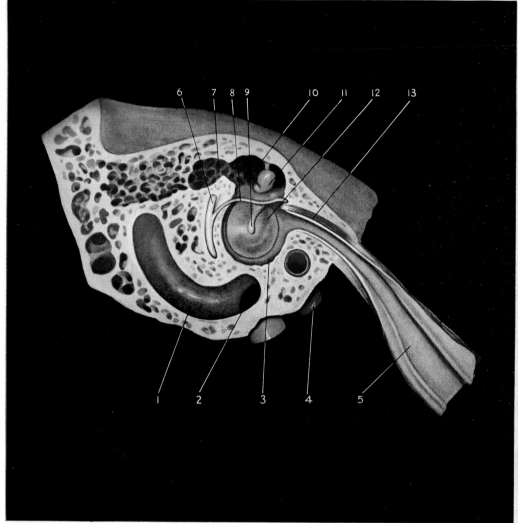

PLATE II

©1946 - AURALGAN - OTOSMOSAN

Middle Ear Viewed from Within

(1) Sigmoid Sinus – (2) Jugular Bulb – (3) Hypotympanum
(4) Internal Carotid Artery – (5) Eustachian Tube – (6) Descending Portion of Facial Nerve – (7) Aditus Ad Antrum
(8) Chord of Tympani Nerve – (9) Hammer Handle – (10)
Epitympanic Space – (11) Head of Malleus – (12) Inner
Aspect of Tympanic Membrane – (13) Tensor Tympanic Muscle

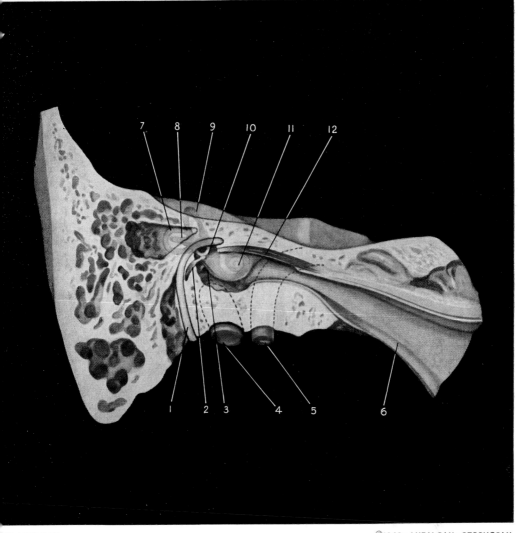

PLATE III

©1946 - AURALGAN - OTOSMOSAN

Inner Wall of Middle Ear

(MEMBRANEOUS LABYRINTH IN TRANSPARENCY)

(1) Facial Nerve — (2) Stapedius Muscle — (3) Round Window
(4) Internal Jugular Vein — (5) Internal Carotid Artery — (6)
Eustachian Tube — (7) Posterior semicircular Canal — (8) Horizontal semicircular Canal — (9) Superior semicircular Canal
(10) Stapes in Oval Window — (11) Cochlea — (12) Tensor
Tympanic Muscle

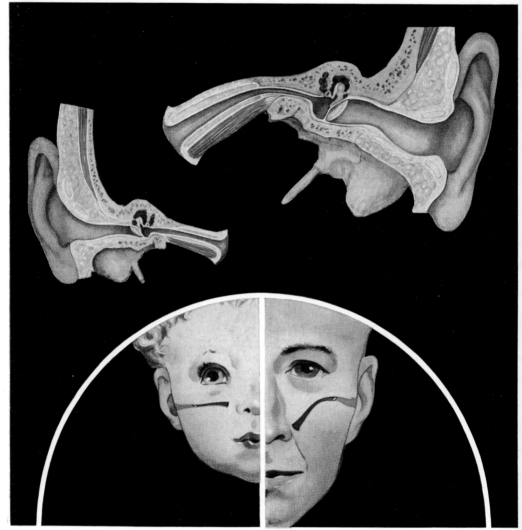

PLATE IV

©1946 - AURALGAN - OTOSMOSAN

Eustachian Tube of Infant and Adult

The infant's tube is straight and patent whereas that of the adult is angulated and closed except during the act of swallowing, yawning, etc. This factor accounts for the frequency of otitis media in early life.

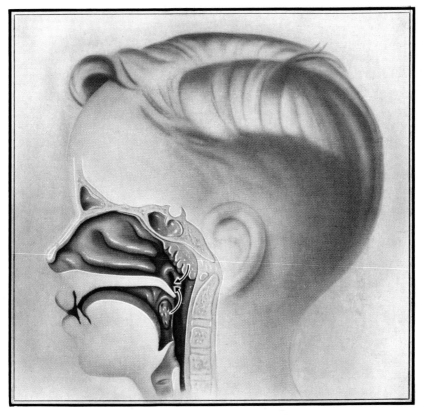

©1946 - AURALGAN - OTOSMOSAN

PLATE IV-A

Sagittal Section of Head of Child

Showing part of Waldeyer's Ring as well as proximity of the
adenoid and the tonsil to the mouth of the Eustachian tube.

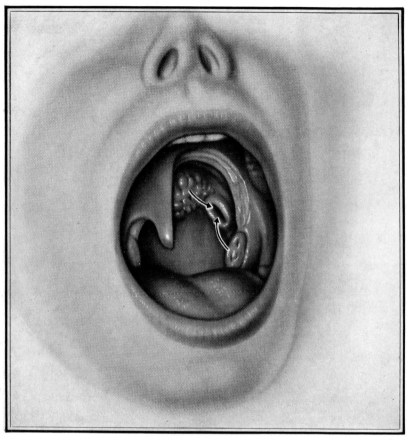

PLATE IV-B   ©1946 - AURALGAN - OTOSMOSAN

Frontal View of Part of Waldeyer's Ring

Showing relationship of tonsil, adenoid and Eustachian tube after removal of one-half of the uvula, soft palate and part of the hard palate on the left side.

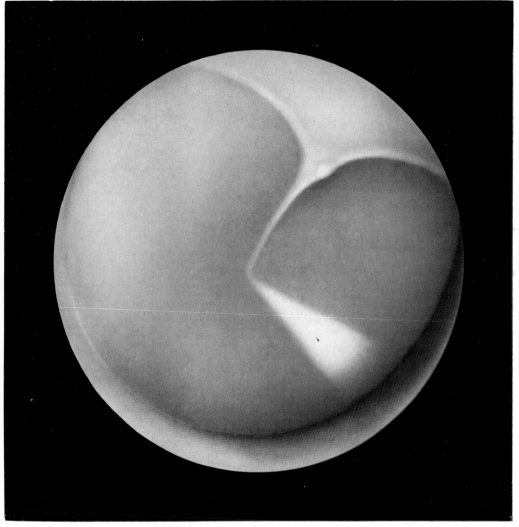

PLATE V
©1946 - AURALGAN - OTOSMOSAN

Normal Tympanic Membrane, Adult
(MEMBRANA TYMPANI)

The color is a dull bluish gray. The landmarks are the long process of the malleus (hammer handle), which terminates about the center of the drum. From this point, called the umbo, a cone of light is seen reflected forward and downward toward the annulus tympanicus. At the upper limit of the hammer handle the short process of the malleus is visible as a teat-like projection. From this point the anterior and posterior fold project laterally and divide the drum into the pars tensa below and the pars flaccida or Shrapnell's membrane above.

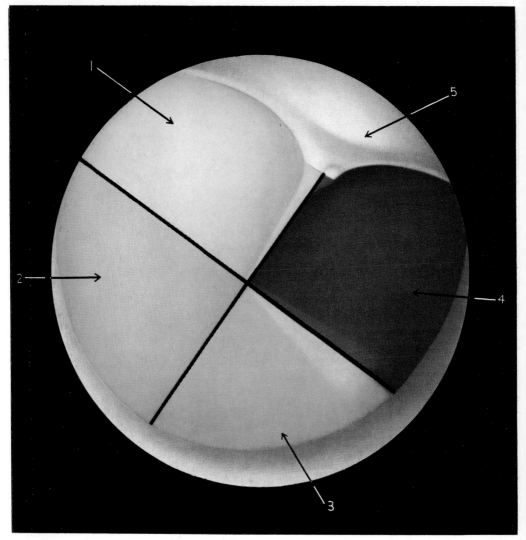

PLATE V-A

©1946 - AURALGAN - OTOSMOSAN

The Quadrants of the Membrana Tympani

(1) Postero-Superior — (2) Postero-Inferior —
(3) Antero-Inferior — (4) Antero-Superior —
(5) Shrapnell's Membrane — not to be considered as
a quadrant. This portion of the drum forms outer wall
of Prussak's space.

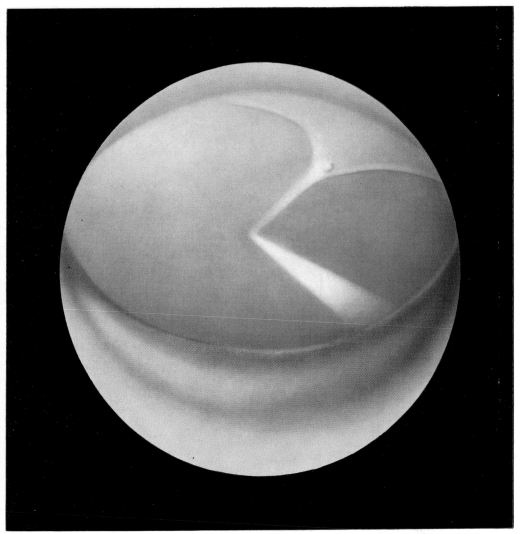

PLATE VI

©1946 - AURALGAN - OTOSMOSAN

Normal Tympanic Membrane, Infant
(MEMBRANA TYMPANI)

The infantile drum presents all the landmarks of the adult drum.
The cone of light however, appears lengthened. Due to the
patent eustachian tube, the drum can be seen to move inward
and outward upon crying and at times with normal respiratory
movement.

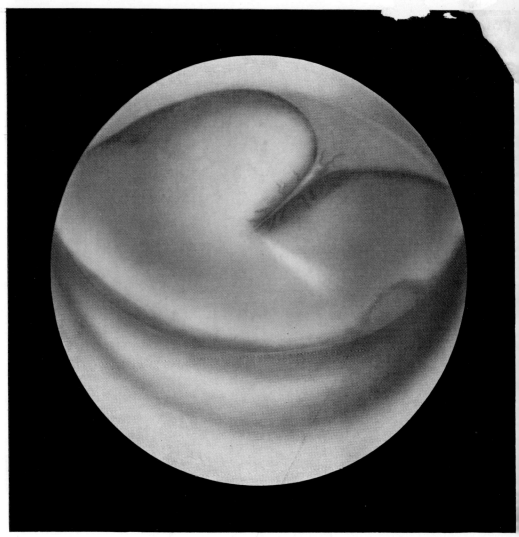

PLATE VII   ©1946 - AURALGAN - OTOSMOSAN

Acute Catarrhal Otitis Media, Infant
(OTITIS MEDIA CATARRHALIS ACUTA NEONATORUM)

May follow any respiratory infection. The redness along the hammer handle, bluish discoloration of Shrapnell's membrane, and engorgement of the vessels in these areas are noted. Redness is frequently present near the annulus tympanicus. The long and short processes are accentuated. The membrana tensa is retracted. The cone of light is foreshortened.

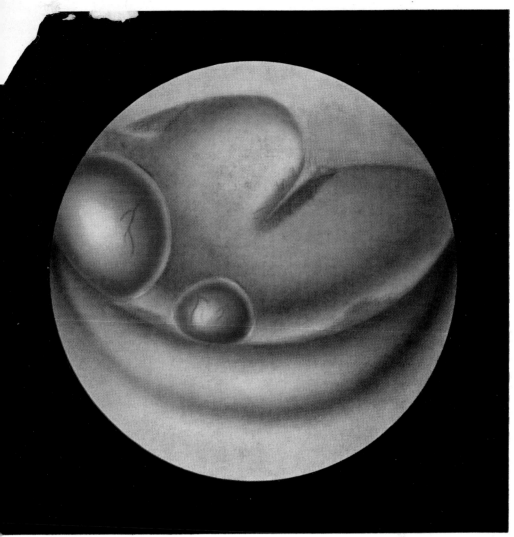

PLATE VIII

©1946 - AURALGAN - OTOSMOSAN

Grippe Otitis, Infant
(OTITIS INFLUENZAE NEONATORUM)
(MYRINGITIS BULLOSA HEMORRHAGICA)

One or more hemorrhagic blebs appear on the surface of the drum. They may be located in any quadrant of the tympanic membrane. They result from extravasation of blood between the outer and middle layers. When present in the postero-superior quadrant they may be mistaken for bulging. The hammer handle, Shrapnell's membrane and other portions of the drum are injected and reddened. These blebs should not be incised.

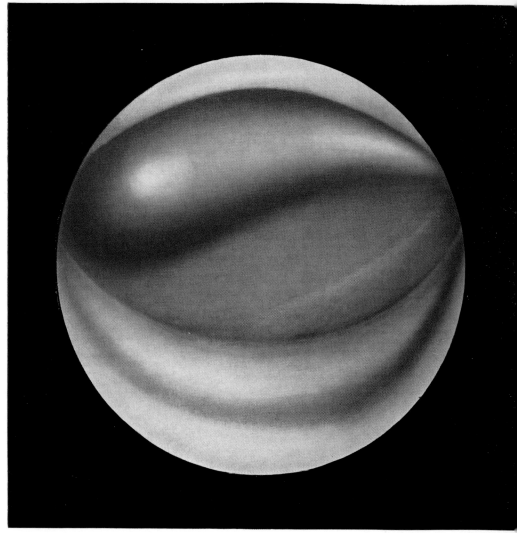

PLATE IX

©1946 - AURALGAN - OTOSMOSAN

Acute Purulent Otitis Media, Infant
(OTITIS MEDIA EXUDATA ACUTA NEONATORUM)
(EARLY STAGE)

The bulging of Shrapnell's membrane and the postero-superior quadrant is evident. All landmarks are obliterated. The antero-inferior quadrant becomes a dullish gray. Pain is an associated symptom. Where this picture results from intra-tympanic congestion it will subside under local palliative therapy.

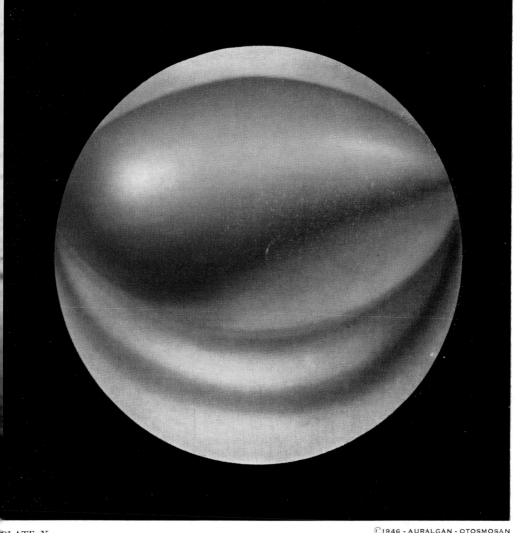

PLATE X

©1946 - AURALGAN - OTOSMOSAN

Acute Purulent Otitis Media, Infant
(OTITIS MEDIA EXUDATA ACUTA NEONATORUM)
(SUPPURATIVE STAGE)

Here the bulging has increased in extent to involve the postero-inferior quadrant. The antero-inferior quadrant also shows signs of inflammatory involvement. This indicates a tympanic empyema. The landmarks here are also absent.

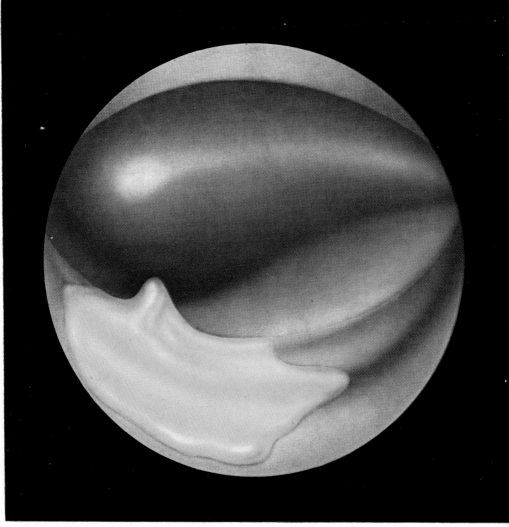

PLATE XI

©1946 - AURALGAN - OTOSMOSAN

Acute Purulent Otitis Media, Infant
(OTITIS MEDIA EXUDATA ACUTA NEONATORUM)
(SPONTANEOUS PERFORATION)

A spontaneous rupture in the infant occurs most frequently in the postero-inferior quadrant. The perforation can be visualized only after the external auditory canal has been thoroughly cleansed of purulent exudate. When perforation occurs pain disappears and fever usually subsides.

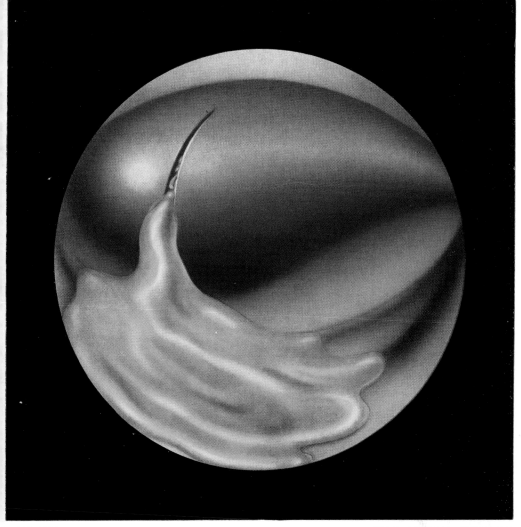

©1946 - AURALGAN - OTOSMOSAN

PLATE XII

Acute Purulent Otitis Media, Infant
(OTITIS MEDIA EXUDATA ACUTA NEONATORUM)
(MYRINGOTOMY; PARACENTESIS)

Immediately following myringotomy pus mixed with blood wells through the incision in the drum. The upper part of the incision heals rapidly and the subsequent otoscopic picture becomes identical with plate No. XI.

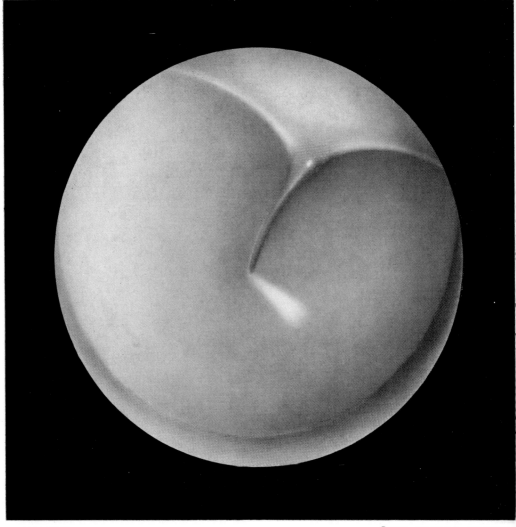

PLATE XIII

©1946 - AURALGAN - OTOSMOSAN

Acute Catarrhal Otitis Media, Adult
(OTITIS MEDIA CATARRHALIS ACUTA)
(FIRST STAGE)

This follows the common cold, sinus infections, and other upper respiratory diseases. The characteristics are injection of the hammer handle and short process and shortening of the light reflex.

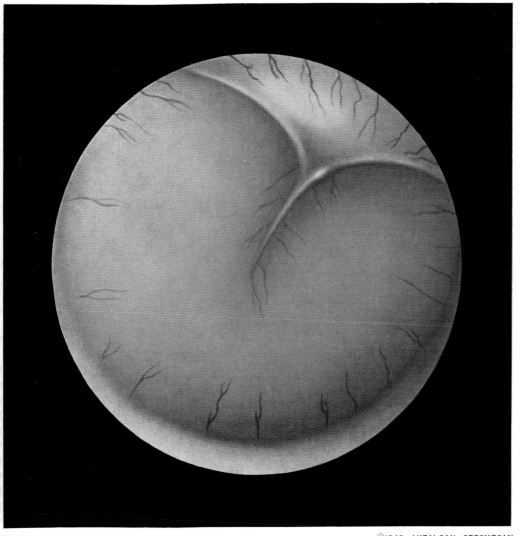

PLATE XIV

©1946 - AURALGAN - OTOSMOSAN

Acute Catarrhal Otitis Media, Adult
(OTITIS MEDIA CATARRHALIS ACUTA)
(SECOND STAGE)

With progression of the lesion the vessels around the periphery of the drum and the long process of the malleus become prominent. There is an increase in the amount of redness, beginning retraction of the entire drum and early accentuation of the short process.

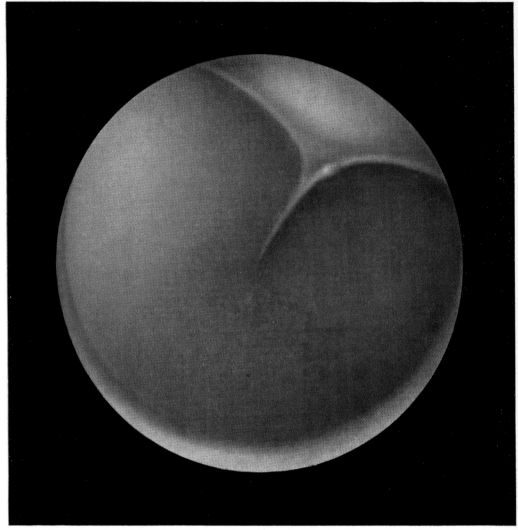

PLATE XV

©1946 - AURALGAN - OTOSMOSAN

Acute Catarrhal Otitis Media, Adult
(OTITIS MEDIA CATARRHALIS ACUTA)
(FINAL STAGE, BEFORE TRANSUDATION)

The entire drum presents a diffuse redness and is markedly retracted. There is increased prominence of the short and long processes. The cone of light is absent. All three stages are associated with the feeling of fullness in the ear and a degree of otalgia.

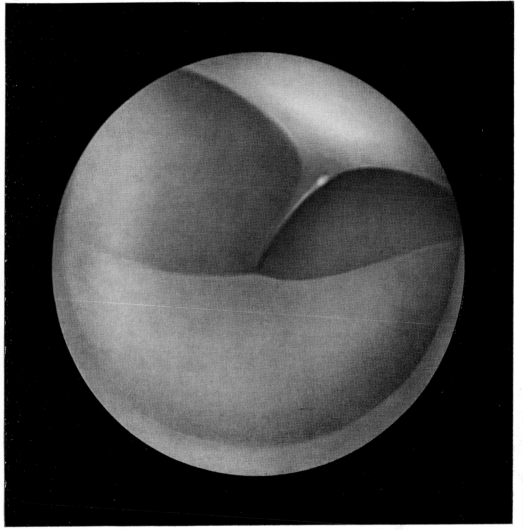

PLATE XVI

©1946 - AURALGAN - OTOSMOSAN

Serous Otitis Media
(OTITIS MEDIA ACUTA TRANSUDATIVA)

A continuance of the catarrhal process results in a serous trans-
udate into the tympanic cavity. A fluid level can be seen at the
height of the umbo. In this stage the inflammatory reaction in
Shrapnell's membrane and in the region of the malleus dimin-
ishes.

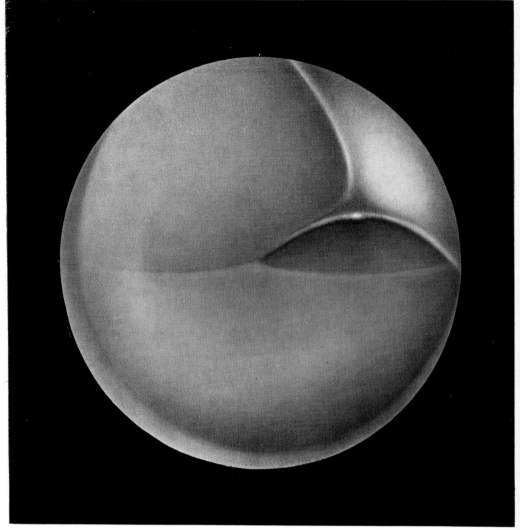

PLATE XVII

©1946 - AURALGAN - OTOSMOSAN

Serous Otitis Media

(OTITIS MEDIA ACUTA TRANSUDATIVA)

Upon tilting the head forward the fluid level is seen to shift with the change in position of the head. This is an important diagnostic sign.

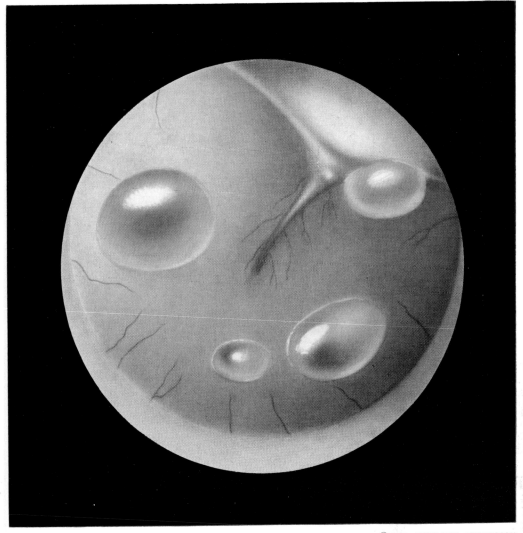

PLATE XVIII

©1946 - AURALGAN - OTOSMOSAN

Bullous Myringitis

(MYRINGITIS BULLOSA SEROSA)

An upper respiratory infection may produce one or more serous blebs underneath the epidermal layer of the drum. They are associated with injection of the hammer handle and the capillaries around the periphery. The remainder of the tympanic membrane is dull but not injected.

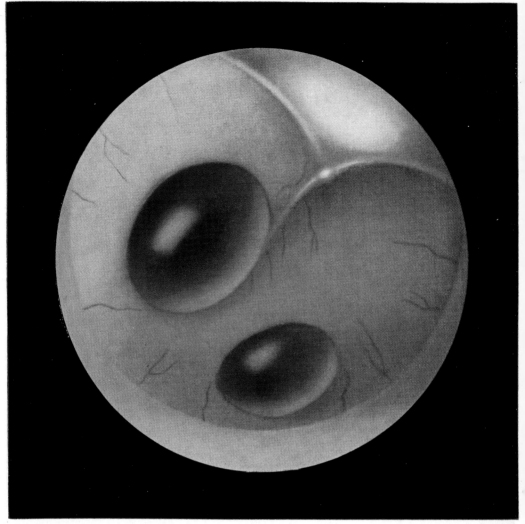

PLATE XIX

©1946 - AURALGAN - OTOSMOSAN

Grippe Otitis Media, Adult
(OTITIS INFLUENZAE)
(MYRINGITIS BULLOSA HEMORRHAGICA)

During an attack of grippe one or more hemorrhagic blebs may appear on the surface beneath the epidermis of the drum. Their association with redness of the rest of the tympanic membrane and accentuation of the landmarks differentiate them from bulging due to purulency.

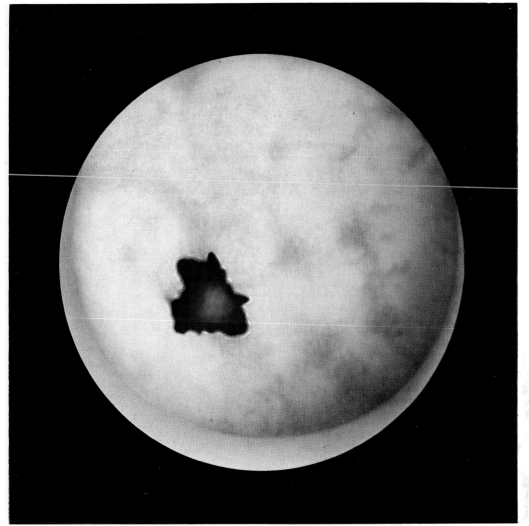

PLATE XX

©1946 - AURALGAN - OTOSMOSAN

Drum Following the Use of Phenol-Glycerin

The use of ear drops containing phenol may lead to extensive scarification and at times necrosis of the drum with a persistent perforation. Milder cases show a continuing redness after the otitis has resolved.

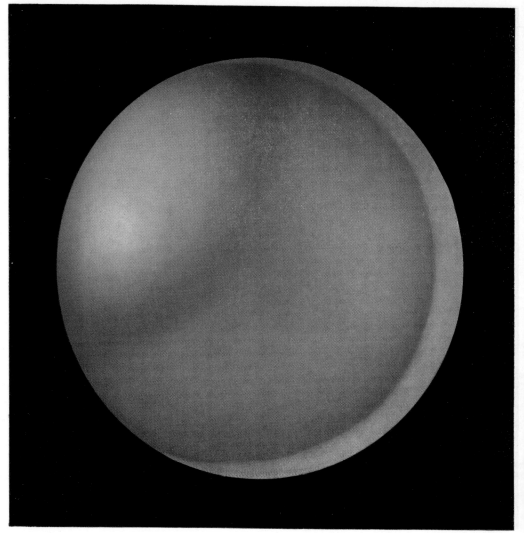

PLATE XXI

©1946 - AURALGAN - OTOSMOSAN

Acute Purulent Otitis Media, Adult

(OTITIS MEDIA PURULENTA ACUTA) (EARLY STAGE)

The first sign of intratympanic suppuration is a moderate bulging in the postero-superior quadrant, a diffuse redness and an absence of landmarks. Where pain is absent myringotomy may be delayed.

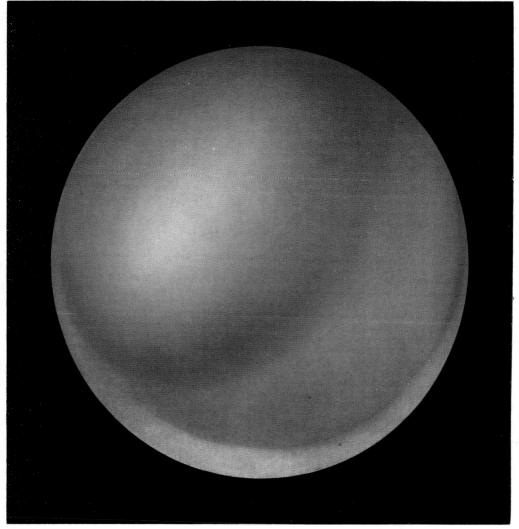

PLATE XXII

©1946 - AURALGAN - OTOSMOSAN

Acute Purulent Otitis Media, Adult
(OTITIS MEDIA PURULENTA ACUTA) (ADVANCED STAGE)

Further progress produces a more marked bulging which at times occupies the entire superior, posterior and inferior quadrants. This otoscopic finding is an indication for myringotomy.

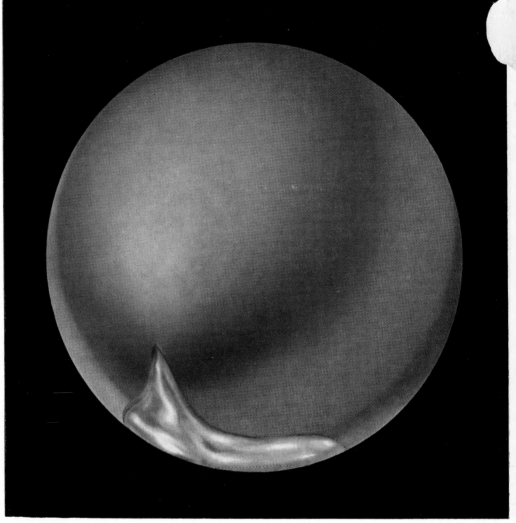

©1946 - AURALGAN - OTOSMOSAN

PLATE XXIII

Acute Purulent Otitis Media, Adult
(OTITIS MEDIA PERFORATA ACUTA)

The most frequent sight of spontaneous perforation is in the postero-inferior quadrant. At first the otoscopic findings show in addition to the otorrhea, a persistence of the bulging.

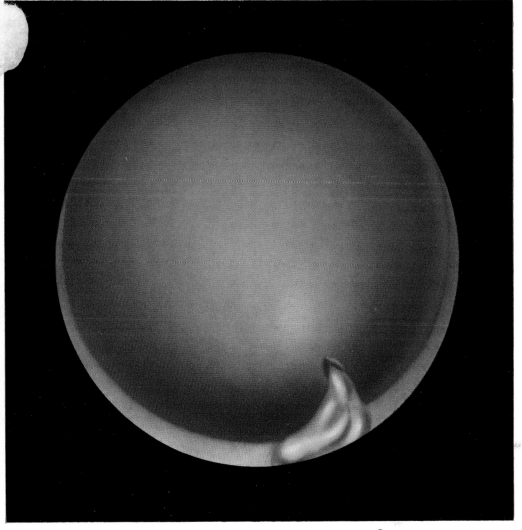

PLATE XXIV

©1946 - AURALGAN - OTOSMOSAN

Acute Purulent Otitis Media, Adult
(OTITIS MEDIA PERFORATA ACUTA)

Where spontaneous rupture occurs in the antero-inferior quadrant the perforation is alluded to as a tubal perforation. It is
meant to convey that the eustachian tube is more severely involved than the middle ear and presages a favorable prognosis.

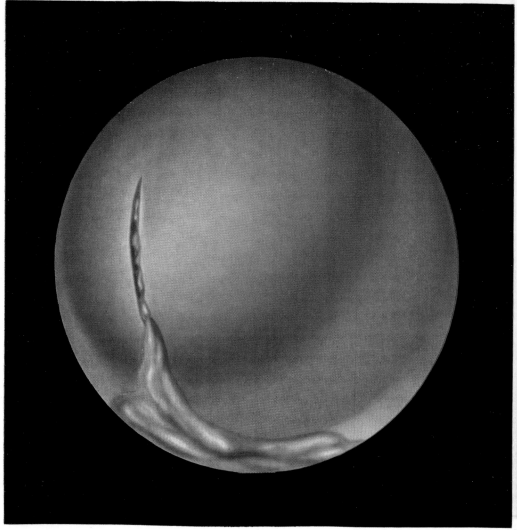

PLATE XXV

©1946 - AURALGAN - OTOSMOSAN

Acute Purulent Otitis Media
(OTITIS MEDIA PURULENTA ACUTA)
(MYRINGOTOMY; PARACENTESIS)

An incision in the tympanic membrane is curvilinear and embraces the postero-superior and postero-inferior quadrants. This is the so-called "area of election," for myringotomy since it affords the optimum in drainage.

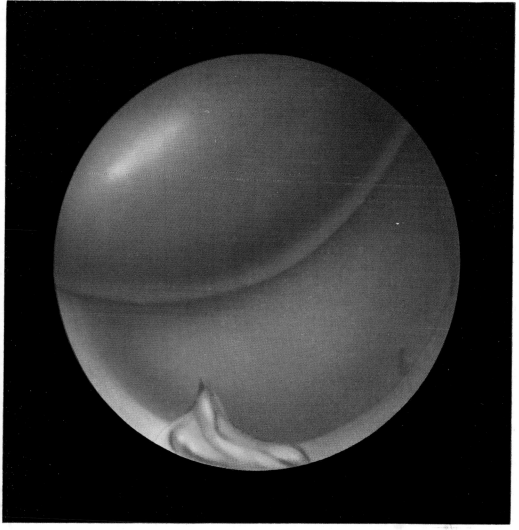

PLATE XXVI

©1946 - AURALGAN - OTOSMOSAN

Acute Coalescent Mastoiditis
(SAGGING OR DROOPING OF SUPERIOR CANAL WALL)

This is one of the earliest signs of coalescent mastoiditis. The edema of the external canal tissues lining the outer attic wall and antrum causes them to protrude down into the canal, thus obliterating from view the upper portion of the drum. This otoscopic picture is sometimes called "narrowing of the fundus."

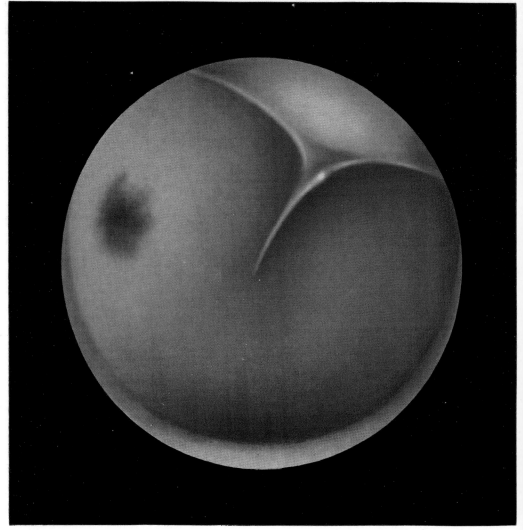

PLATE XXVII

©1946 - AURALGAN - OTOSMOSAN

Aero-Otitis, (The Blocked Ear)
(FIRST DEGREE)

Changes in air pressure such as occur in aviation and caisson work are the causes. The entire tympanic membrane is reddened and retracted. The landmarks are accentuated. A hemorrhage between the layers of the drum is noted in the postero-superior quadrant.

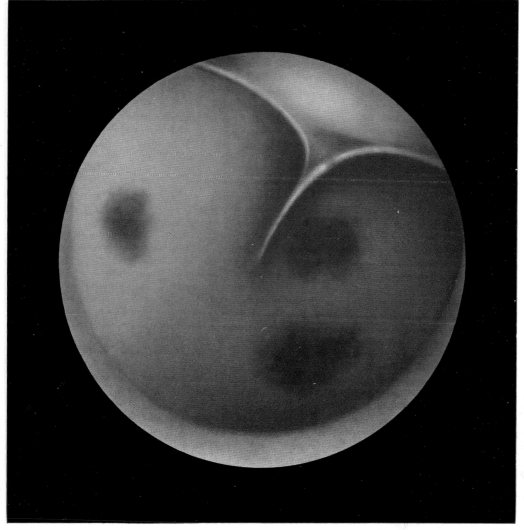

PLATE XXVIII

©1946 - AURALGAN - OTOSMOSAN

Aero-Otitis, (The Blocked Ear)
(FIRST DEGREE)

Multiple hemorrhages are not infrequent with this stage. The loss in hearing acuity following this trauma is surprisingly little. With proper therapy hearing is returned to normal.

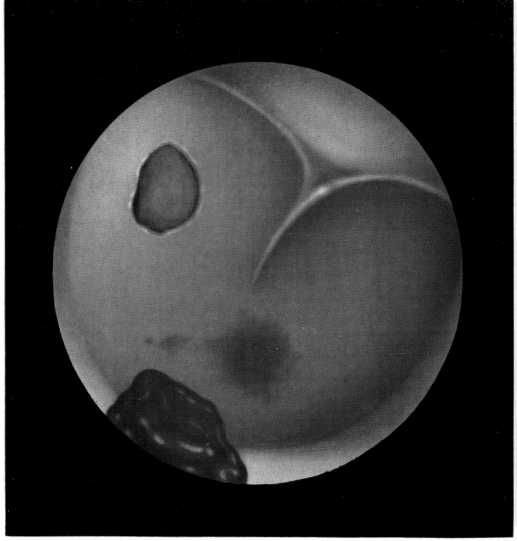

PLATE XXIX

©1946 - AURALGAN - OTOSMOSAN

Aero-Otitis, (The Blocked Ear)

(TRAUMATIC RUPTURE)

Immediate inspection reveals a ragged perforation of the membrana tympani, situated most frequently in the postero-superior quadrant, and a coagulum of blood in the external canal. Perforations may be multiple. They are almost always associated with one or more hemorrhages in the drum substance.

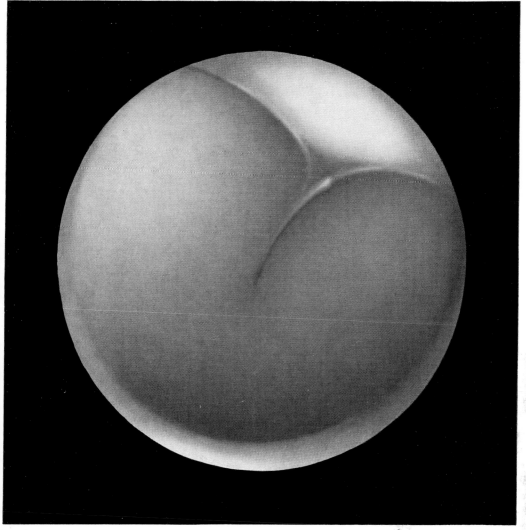

PLATE XXX

©1946 - AURALGAN - OTOSMOSAN

Aero-Otitis, (The Blocked Ear)
(INTRATYMPANIC HEMORRHAGE)

Severe alteration in air pressure may produce an intratympanic hemorrhage. This is seen otoscopically as a bluish translucence through the drum. The hammer handle and short process are injected. Isolated hemorrhages in the drum itself may also accompany this picture.

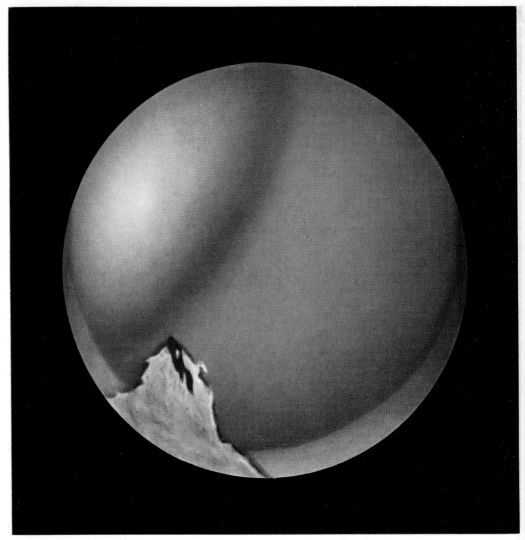

PLATE XXXI

©1946 - AURALGAN - OTOSMOSAN

Diphtheritic Otitis Media

The tympanic membrane shows a mild inflammatory involvement. Through the perforation a thin serous discharge exudes.
The margins of the perforation are covered with a dirty gray
membrane. Attempt to remove this membrane is followed by
bleeding.

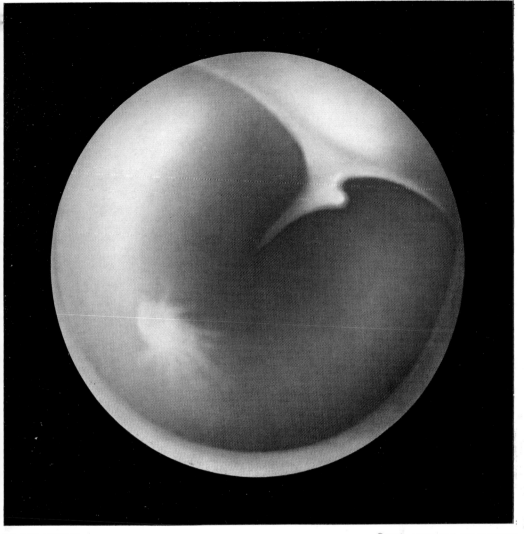

PLATE XXXII

©1946 - AURALGAN - OTOSMOSAN

Chronic Catarrhal Otitis Media
(CALCAREOUS DEPOSITS)

In the chronic catarrhal otitis media of long standing and in the reparative process following perforation of the drum, calcium deposits are frequently seen. They represent the end result of repair.

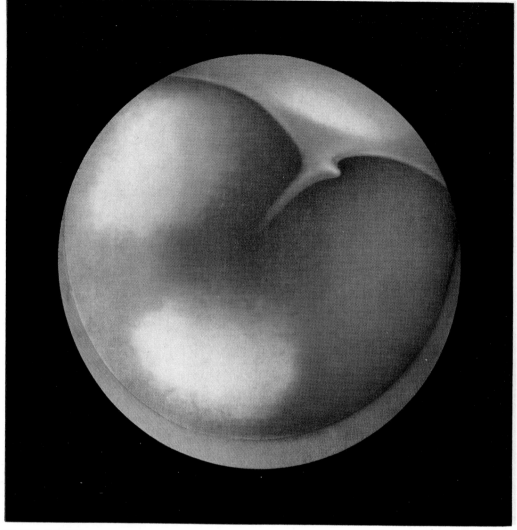

PLATE XXXIII ©1946 - AURALGAN - OTOSMOSAN

Chronic Catarrhal Otitis Media
(OTITIS MEDIA CATARRHALIS CHRONICA)

The entire drum is markedly retracted and all landmarks distorted and accentuated due to intratympanic adhesions. The color is a dull gray.

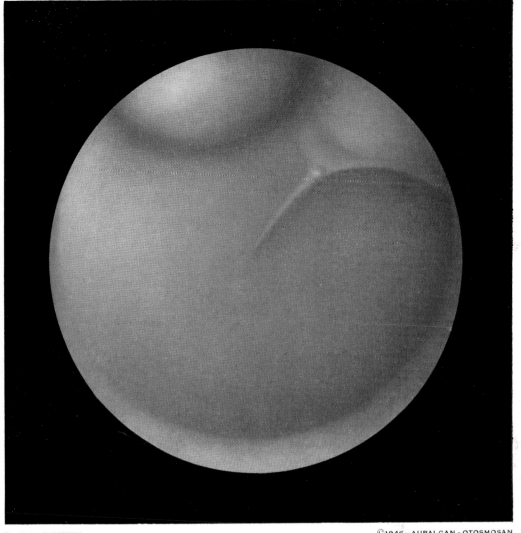

PLATE XXXIV

©1946 - AURALGAN - OTOSMOSAN

Acute Necrotic Otitis Media
(OTITIS MEDIA NECROTICA ACUTA)
(SCARLATINAL OTITIS MEDIA)

This occurs most frequently during the early period of scarlet fever. The earliest stage shows a slight bulge involving the upper portion of the drum and includes Shrapnell's membrane. The remainder of the drum is reddened but the landmarks are visible.

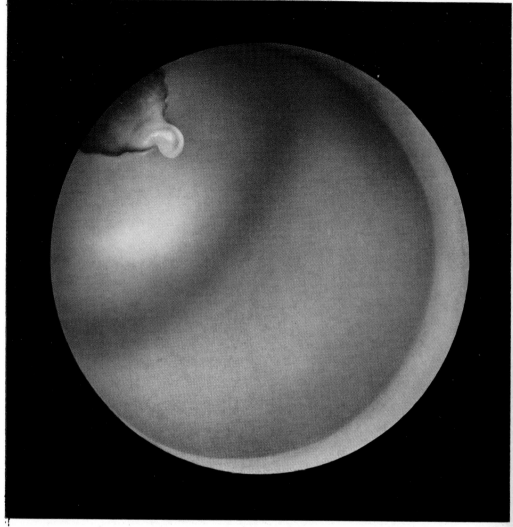

PLATE XXXV

©1946 - AURALGAN - OTOSMOSAN

Acute Necrotic Otitis Media
(OTITIS MEDIA NECROTICA ACUTA)
(SCARLATINAL OTITIS MEDIA)

The next stage which may appear within a few hours shows a
marginal erosion of the drum usually postero-superiorly and
a scanty purulent discharge. The drum itself beyond the slight
bulge shows little inflammatory reaction.

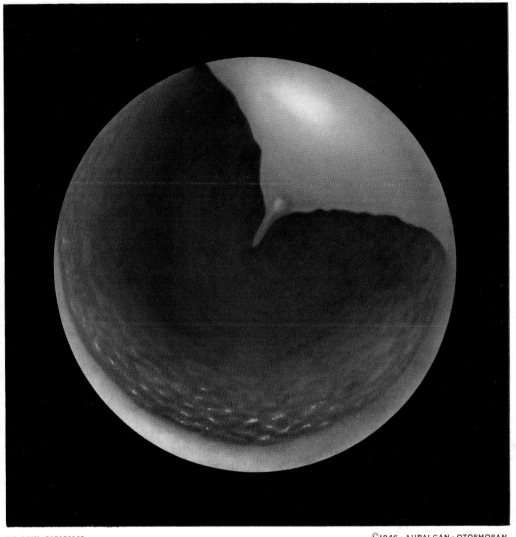

PLATE XXXVI

©1946 - AURALGAN - OTOSMOSAN

Acute Necrotic Otitis Media
(OTITIS MEDIA NECROTICA ACUTA)
(SCARLATINAL OTITIS MEDIA)

Within a short period, at times less than a day, the entire pars tensa is destroyed. The tympanic mucosa is also destroyed. The long process of the malleus is involved in the mass necrosis. Otoscopy shows an angry granulating middle ear, where only remnants of the drum persist. Seen years later this condition is the "Chronic Purulent Otitis Media Due to Bone Necrosis."

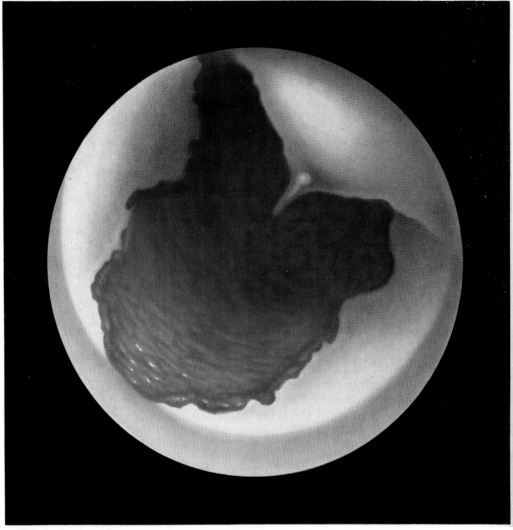

PLATE XXXVII

©1946 - AURALGAN - OTOSMOSAN

Acute Necrotic Otitis Media
(OTITIS MEDIA NECROTICA ACUTA)
(SCARLATINAL OTITIS MEDIA, REPARATIVE PROCESS)

Nature's attempt at repair is the ingrowth of epidermis from the external canal through the marginal perforation so as to blanket the granulating surface in the middle ear with a cloak of epithelium. This is the primary stage of a "pseudocholesteatoma."

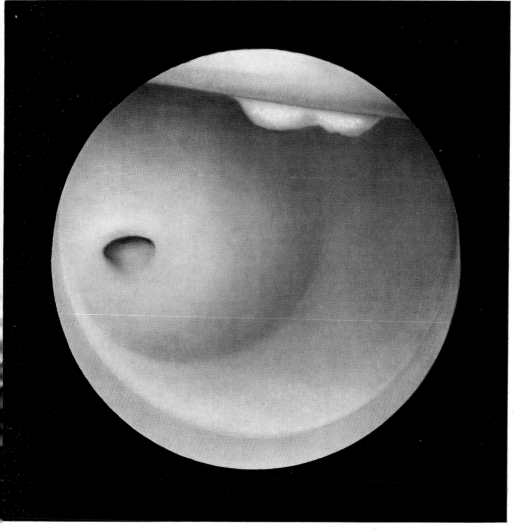

PLATE XXXVIII

©1946 - AURALGAN - OTOSMOSAN

Pseudocholesteatoma

A fully developed pseudocholesteatoma shows the entire drum including Shrapnell's membrane to be absent. The inner tympanic wall is lined by grayish epidermis. Behind the bony attic wall above, cholesteatome masses are seen protruding from the epitympanic space. The round window and the promontory are visible.

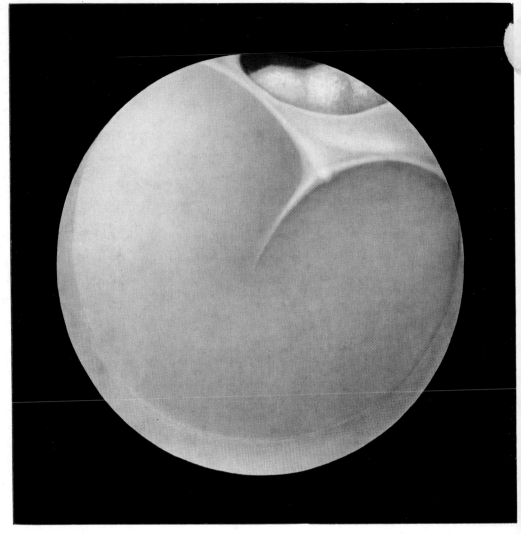

©1946 - AURALGAN - OTOSMOSAN

PLATE XXXIX

Cholesteatoma (Attic Perforation)

Where a perforation has occurred in Shrapnell's membrane a
cholesteatoma may form leaving the remainder of the tympanic
membrane intact and normal in appearance.

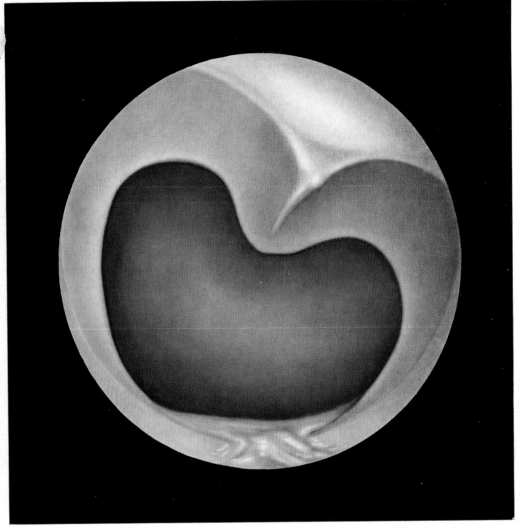

PLATE XL

©1946 - AURALGAN - OTOSMOSAN

Chronic Purulent Otitis Media (non-dangerous)

(OTITIS MEDIA PURULENTA CHRONICA)

This is due to a chronic suppuration of the tympanic mucosa.
A kidney shaped perforation is the most common one. Any type
perforation may occur but some drum tissue between the
annulus and the defect is always present.

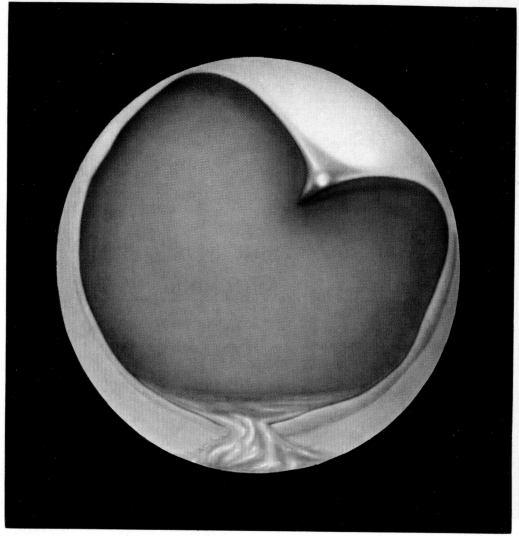

PLATE XLI

©1946 - AURALGAN - OTOSMOSAN

Chronic Purulent Otitis Media (non-dangerous)

(OTITIS MEDIA PURULENTA CHRONICA)

Here a central type perforation occupies the entire pars tensa. Note drum tissue remaining between annulus and the tympanic defect. The malleus is adherent to the inner tympanic wall. This type of chronicity (also plate No. XL) requires no surgery to the temporal bone.

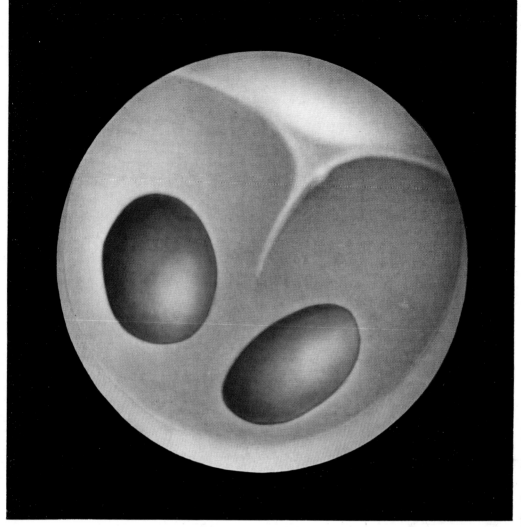

©1946 - AURALGAN - OTOSMOSAN

PLATE XLII

Multiple Perforations

Where the pars tensa is otherwise intact and no otorrhea is
present and landmarks are visible, multiple perforations should
suggest trauma, particularly that resulting from gun fire.

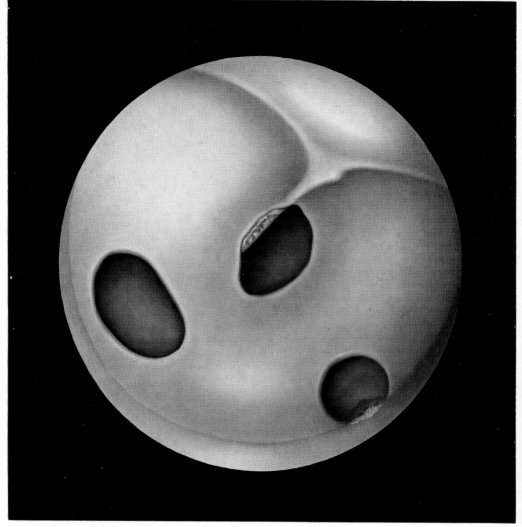

PLATE XLIII

©1946 - AURALGAN - OTOSMOSAN

Tuberculous Otitis Media

Where perforations are multiple and are associated with otor-

rhea, a tuberculosis of the middle ear should be suspected. These

perforations result from breaking down of tubercles.

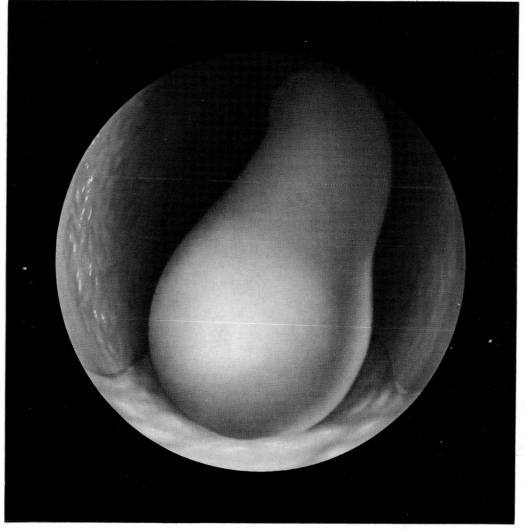

PLATE XLIV

©1946 - AURALGAN - OTOSMOSAN

Aural Polyps

Aural polyps are usually the result of a chronic purulent otitis media of the dangerous type and indicate bone necrosis. They may protrude through any portion of the drum, and frequently are of such size as to obstruct full visualization of the fundus.

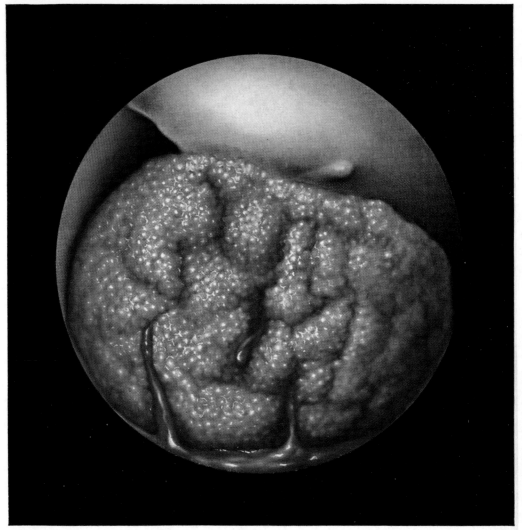

PLATE XLV © 1946 - AURALGAN - OTOSMOSAN

Malignancy of Middle Ear

A tumor growth should be suspected when the polypoid mass bleeds profusely when touched. This distinguishes it from an aural polyp due to bone necrosis. Positive diagnosis is made by biopsy.

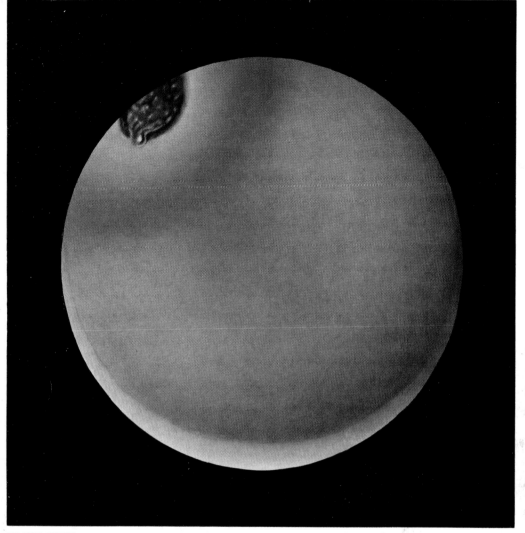

PLATE XLVI

©1946 - AURALGAN - OTOSMOSAN

Syphilis of the Middle Ear

Occurs in the tertiary stage. It appears as a protrusion of the
postero-superior quadrant and posterior canal wall associated
with a thin watery discharge and loss of hearing. Incision yields
no pus; pain is absent. Positive diagnosis by serological tests.

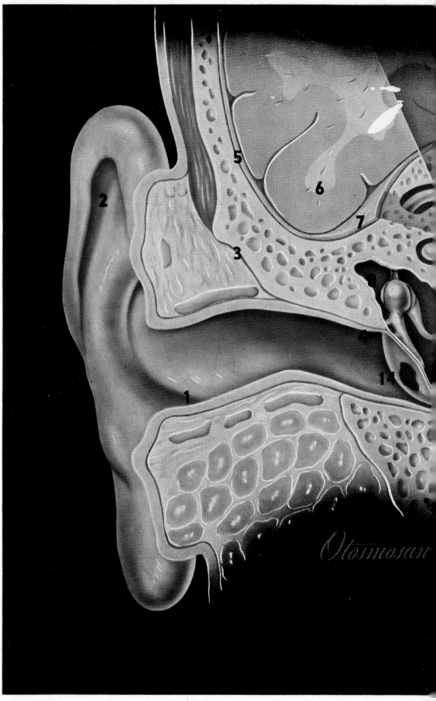

PLATE XLVII

Some locations of severe and grave lesio

(1) Circumscribed furuncle of otitis externa — (2) Infection of the cartilage of concha. (External ear.) — (3) Subperiosteal collection of pus in case of perforated cortex. (Subperiosteal abscess.) — (4) Sinking of post-superior canal wall, during periosteal inflammation, as part of picture of acute mastoiditis — (5) Epidural cerebral abscess — (6) Circumscribed cerebral abscess — (7) Subdural abscess — (8) Cholesteatoma (pseudo) situated in the attic of middle ear — (9) Circumscribed

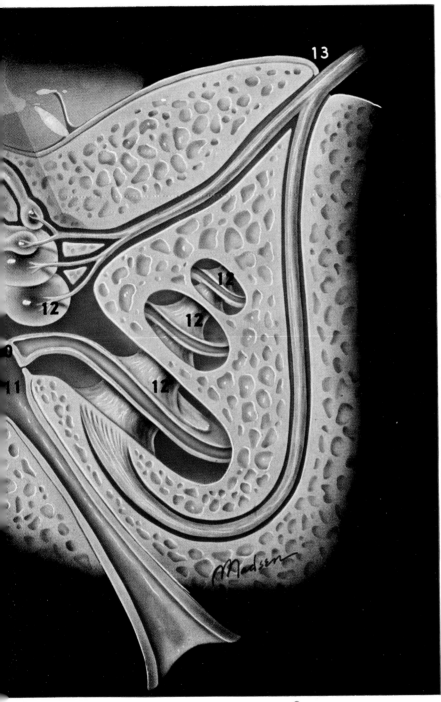

© 1946 - AURALGAN — OTOSMOSAN

nd their sites, diagrammatically indicated.

labyrinthitis — (10) Calcareous deposits cause ankylosis of stapes, involving the annular ligament — (11) Fistula opening on roof of tympanic orifice of Eustachian tube leading to disease in petrosal pyramid — (12) When these areas are involved, the labyrinth is the seat of the lesion — (13) By pressure on the auditory nerve, especially its vestibular branches, symptoms of an angle tumor become evident — (14) Perforated ear drum

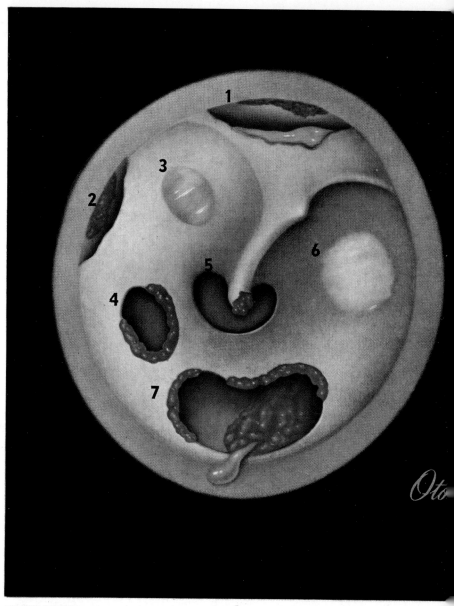

PLATE XLVIII

Composite Illustrations of Tympanic Membrane
in Chron
FIRST DRUM

(1) Perforation of Shrapnel's membrane with bone erosion and pus — (2) Marginal perforation with bone erosion — (3) Healed perforation with regenerated drum membrane — (4) Granulations on an irregular perforation — (5) Ossicular necrosis — kidney-shaped perforation — (6) Calcified scar tissue — (7) Granulations and pus — eustachian tube infection

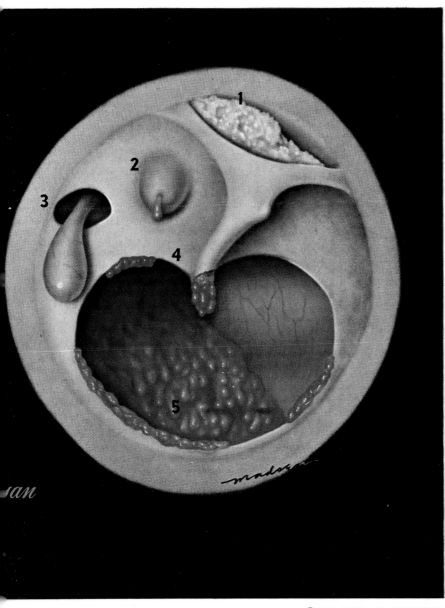

©1946 - AURALGAN - OTOSMOSAN

owing Various Types of Pathology and Perforations
ppurating Ears.   SECOND DRUM

(1) Cholesteatoma seen through perforation in Shrapnel's membrane — (2) Nipple-
like perforation — (3) Polyp protruding through perforation — (4) Granulations
and bone necrosis of the ossicle — (5) Granulations on promontory and along
margins of perforation

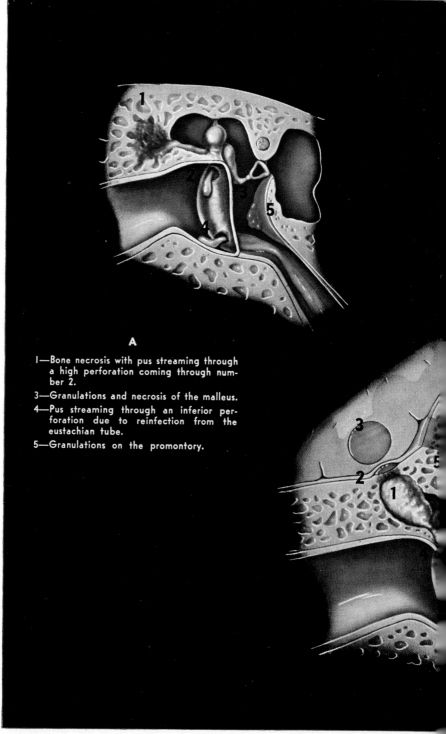

A

1—Bone necrosis with pus streaming through a high perforation coming through number 2.

3—Granulations and necrosis of the malleus.

4—Pus streaming through an inferior perforation due to reinfection from the eustachian tube.

5—Granulations on the promontory.

PLATE XLIX

Some locations of severe and grave com

Diagramm

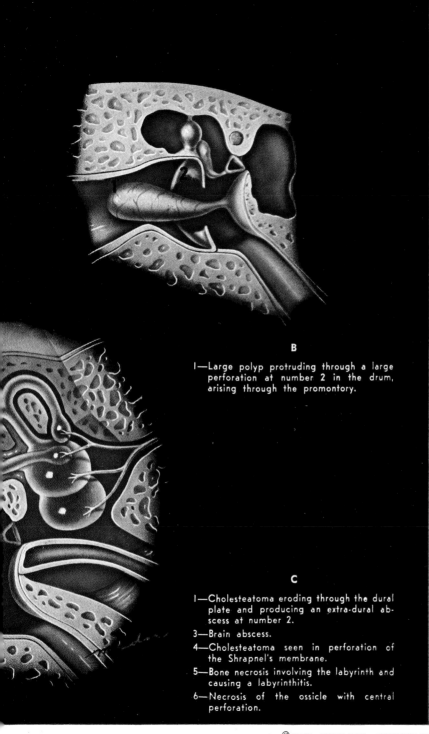

B

1—Large polyp protruding through a large perforation at number 2 in the drum, arising through the promontory.

C

1—Cholesteatoma eroding through the dural plate and producing an extra-dural abscess at number 2.

3—Brain abscess.

4—Cholesteatoma seen in perforation of the Shrapnel's membrane.

5—Bone necrosis involving the labyrinth and causing a labyrinthitis.

6—Necrosis of the ossicle with central perforation.

© 1946 - AURALGAN — OTOSMOSAN

ions of chronic suppurative Otitis Media,

y indicated.

Visual Education in Otology

A Library of 16 mm. Sound and Color Films, available for booking to medical societies, hospitals, universities and physician study-groups of 20 or more professional persons in attendance . . . gratis, with the compliments of the makers of Auralgan.

AVAILABLE WITHOUT CHARGE — Film, projector, sound equipment, screen and competent operator are supplied wherever such facilities are not available.

BOOK EARLY! — The unprecedented demand for these eight visual education films is so great that bookings should be made at least three weeks in advance with indication of alternate date.

Subjects

1. The Anatomy of the Ear
2. Otoscopy in the Inflammations
3. Otitis Media in Pediatrics
4. A Clinic on Acute Mastoiditis
5. A Clinic on Chronic Otitic Purulencies
6. A Dry Clinic on Sinus Thrombosis
7. Suppurative Petrositis, Meningeal
8. Clinic on the Deafened

Running time approximately 30 minutes.

These and other films now being made are produced under the able direction and supervision of eminent otologists.

AURALGAN RESEARCH DIVISION
New York, N. Y.

Colored Lantern Slides

. . . depicting the Anatomical and Pathological Conditions of the Ear. This complete set of 36 slides available without charge for instruction of nurses, physician study groups, university instructors, accredited medical societies, hospital staffs.

These slides are loaned gratis to the above listed groups possessing their own projection facilities.

Subjects

1. Frontal Section Through Tympanic Cavity
2. Middle Ear Viewed from Within
3. Inner Wall of Middle Ear
4. Eustachian Tube of Infant and Adult
5. Sagittal Section of Head of Child
6. Frontal View, of Part of Waldeyer's Ring
7. The Quadrants of the Membrana Tympani
8. Normal Tympanic Membrane, Infant
9. Grippe Otitis, Infant
10. Acute Purulent Otitis Media, Infant
11. Normal Tympanic Membrane, Adult
12. Acute Catarrhal Otitis Media (1st Stage)
13. Acute Catarrhal Otitis Media (2nd Stage)
14. Acute Catarrhal Otitis Media, Adult (Final)
15. Drum Following the Use of Phenol-Glycerin
16. Acute Purulent Otitis Media, Adult (Advanced)
17. Acute Purulent Otitis Media (Spont. Perf.)
18. Acute Purulent Otitis Media (Paracentesis)
19. Serous Otitis Media
20. Bullous Myringitis
21. Grippe Otitis Media, Adult
22. Acute Coalescent Mastoiditis
23. Aero-Otitis (1st degree)
24. Aero-Otitis (Traumatic Rupture)
25. Aero-Otitis (Intratympanic Hemorrhage)
26. Chronic Catarrhal Otitis Media
27. Acute Necrotic Otitis Media (Scarlatinal)
28. Acute Necrotic Otitis Media (Reparative Process)
29. Cholesteatoma (Attic Perforation)
30. Chronic Purulent Otitis Media (non-dangerous)
31. Malignancy of Middle Ear
32. Multiple Perforations
33. Aural Polyps
34. Syphilis of the Middle Ear
35. Tuberculous Otitis Media
36. Diphtheritic Otitis Media

AURALGAN RESEARCH DIVISION
New York, N. Y.